CHRIS GRIFFITHS

Fasting and Fitness

Unlocking a healthier you

Disclaimer

I hope you the readers are inspired by what I did to overcome my health struggles.

Before attempting any new fasting and fitness regime, please speak to your doctor or physician so that they can carry out any relevant medical tests and examinations before you commence any new fasting and fitness regime.

I would recommend that you do not attempt any fitness and fasting regime until your doctor or physician has given you the green light to start.

First edition

Contents

1

Introduction

Unlocking a Healthier You Without Sacrificing Enjoyment

Have you ever found yourself caught in the endless loop of diets and meal plans, only to feel frustrated and disheartened when the results fall short or just don't work?

If so, you're not alone.

In the labyrinth of sugary indulgences and failed diets, I stand before you, not just as an author, but as someone who has walked the same path, navigating the confusing world of weight loss and fitness. This book, "Fasting and Fitness," is born out of my struggle with finding a sustainable path to a healthier lifestyle without sacrificing enjoyment.

In my younger days, I was very sporty and participated in daily activities whether working out in the gym, swimming, or playing tennis. As you progress and life takes over you are not as active and you start putting on a few pounds. After years of experimenting with various diets, I discovered a different approach that helped me to shed those extra pounds and helped me to create a positive relationship between food and exercise.

In the pages that follow, I'll share with you the insights and lessons I've learned along my journey in the last twelve months that I used to unlock a healthier me. This isn't just another diet book, it's an insight into the necessary changes and lifestyle shifts that I had to make that allowed me to achieve my fitness goals without sacrificing the joy of eating.

In the labyrinth of sugary indulgences and failed diets, I stand before you, not just as an author, but as someone who has walked the same path, navigating the confusing world of weight loss and fitness. "Fasting and Fitness" is my testament to my triumph after years of personal struggle, procrastination, and doing the wrong things for me whilst being on the roller coaster of ineffective diets. For too long I found myself entangled in the seductive promises of quick fixes – from milkshake regimes to meatless diets, and the glitter and attraction of so-called one-tablet wonders fat-burning tablets. The harsh reality was none of them worked for me. The only thing I did lose was time and money. Frustration became my companion, and the lean body I yearned for seemed like an elusive dream when I looked at my pot belly.

So why should you pick up this book?

This isn't just another compilation of generic advice. The aim of "Fasting and Fitness" is to speak directly to those who, like me, have danced between various diets, caught in the cycle of sugar-laden temptations, this book is your guide to breaking free. But here's the best part: You won't have to bid farewell to the pleasures of eating and drinking, far from it, this is not about full-on deprivation. It is about regaining your self-control, shedding those extra pounds, trimming your waistline, and embracing a healthier you, a more active you, without sacrificing the food and drinks we all love.

Over the past year, I've amassed a treasure trove of knowledge based on my failures and more importantly, the stuff that worked. The most liberating part is that it is all here, in these pages, waiting for you.

I hope that the cost of this book is a small investment in your quest to unlock a healthier you.

Join me on this journey and learn what I had to do to redefine my relationship with food, stop procrastinating, and reclaim my fitness and vitality that was mine to rightfully claim once I had figured out what needed to be done. The experience and lessons I learned allowed me to turn around my blood sugars from pre-diabetic and back to normal in seven months.

In the realm of everyday existence, I am no different from most people with a family. I have a partner, two sons, and a life filled with the ebb and flow of routine and a 9 to 5 job however, there came a point where the reflection in the mirror and the numbers on the weighing scale told a different tale. At my peak, I weighed 92 kilograms, with a 36-inch waist, and a pot belly as an unwelcome badge of honor. I knew looking at my pot belly that something drastic had to change and the pot belly's days were numbered.

Chapter 1: My Story and Diabetes

The Starting Point

The wake-up call came in the form of routine blood sugar test results. I was expecting the results to be fine with nothing to worry about. I had a 36-inch waist and a pot belly that had crept up on me from nowhere. The blood test revealed my worst nightmare. It was a stark revelation that shook me to the core. I was pre-diabetic and staring at the possibility of a future overshadowed by diabetes and everything that comes with diabetes. My mind began to spin with fear and the realization that this was a pivotal moment in my life that could and would alter the course of my life forever.

At that critical moment after I had been hit by one hell of a curve ball, as life sometimes throws at you, I faced a stark choice, accept the consequences of having a high blood sugar count and teetering on having full-blown diabetes or pull my head out of the sand and take responsibility for my health after all I only had myself to blame for getting into this mess in the first place and I owed it to myself and my loved ones to get myself out of this mess.

The Reality Check

I weighed 92 kilograms, harbored a 36-inch waist, and wore a pot belly as an unwelcome badge of honor which I could not shift and showed no signs of wanting to leave me.

Being labeled as pre-diabetic was my stark reality check. It was the harsh whisper of a wake-up call that propelled me into action. No longer could I procrastinate; the fight of my life had just begun. This chapter unfolds the raw and honest narrative of my journey, marked by a daunting starting point, introspective moments in front of the mirror, the weight of responsibility, and the unfiltered reality check that fueled my transformation. This was a big reality check and I had to stand, look it in the eye, and battle with this diagnosis and the implications that followed.

Chapter 2: The Journey Begins

Back to Basics

The turning point was not just about shedding pounds; it was a mental shift, a commitment to rewriting the narrative of my life and taking back control of what I eat and when.

I had to go back to basics, back to the foundational principles that became the purpose of my new determination to implement change. Going back to basics wasn't just a physical act, it was a reboot of my mentality, eating habits, exercise program and my self-control. This was a full-time commitment to reclaim control over my health and my life.

You Are What You Eat

To start the commitment I had to rewrite the narrative of my life. In the labyrinth of dietary trends, I discovered a fundamental truth – our bodies mirror what we consume. Staring at my pot belly made me realize the profound impact that my food choices had made on my well-being and my pot belly. My choice was no longer just about calories, it was about rethinking my way of life so that I was able to nourish my body with the right fuel. Understanding this simple yet powerful concept became the cornerstone of my journey.

Food is integral to everything, your survival and your recovery following exercise. The key to this is eating the right foods and not just eating fast food, takeaway and pizza every day. The foods that are traditionally labeled as "fast foods" can still be eaten but should be done at the weekend and in moderation but only if you have earned it as a reward for all of the effort, and determination it takes to avoid all of the sugar lust of cakes and cookies during the week.

Let me be candid, no law says that you cannot indulge yourself at the weekend with friends and family, have a glass of wine, beers, cakes, and cookies. I quickly realized that provided you have avoided "fast foods" and resisted those urges to indulge in sugar lust during the week, at the weekend it was party time and you had to enjoy yourself as you think fit. When Monday comes it is back to business and the "fast food" and sugar lust are put on hold, until the next weekend.

Portion Size

A revelation as simple as the size of the plate matters. Yes, size does matter. The often-overlooked aspect of portion control plays a massive part in getting your food intake and diet right. I discovered that a little adjustment in the quantity of what's on your plate can be a game-changer in your quest for a healthier you. It's not about deprivation, it is about responsible, measured consumption and savoring every last bite right to the end.

The reduction in your portion sizes is not just about shedding pounds, it is a commitment to rewriting the narrative of my life to unlock a healthier me.

Portion size helps you to maintain a healthy weight and it is well known that if you eat too much and do little or no exercise you will put on weight and your size will increase. If you eat smaller portions and engage in some exercise your weight and size will eventually start to decrease in size.

This was an obstacle and a challenge that I had to engage in because there could only be one winner and that had to be me. I made up my that I would stand, look my diagnosis in the eye, and do battle with this diagnosis.

My Cheat Codes

In the vibrant tapestry of balanced meals and health-conscious foods, salads stand head and shoulder above most foods in my experience. The significance of incorporating salads and green vegetables into my mealtime routine making was crucial in my quest to unlock a healthier me.

Salads and green vegetables are nature's version of the cheat code in a video game. Salads and green vegetables are generously packed with essential vitamins which are the nutrients that are the body's fuel. Salads and green vegetables support good health and can help to provide you with all the ingredients needed to get fit and healthy.

Salads and green vegetables are overlooked, and not eaten enough by people. I decided to include salads and green vegetables every day as part of my food consumption.

Vegetables are fiber and the more fiber you can eat helps to promote a balanced diet. I found that salads and vegetables helped my body digest my food better and promoted regular bowel movements.

I preferred to eat my salad and green vegetables as part of my main meal with a homemade salad dressing comprising of at least apple cider vinegar, a dash of lemon and lime juice, salt and pepper to season. I ate Salads and green vegetables every day without fail.

Salads and green vegetables helped me to feel full and satisfied. Salads stopped me from craving sweet sugary things to the extent that now I cannot eat candy anymore because it simply tastes too sweet for my liking.

Hydration

Hydration is a key element of unlocking a healthier you. The human body is composed of over 50% water which confirms the importance of something that we all have access to. Water and fluids are vital to keep the human body hydrated and can lead to a healthier you.

I found that water was essential for me. The combination of salads, water, and exercise reduced my wind and gas. I found that if my body was properly hydrated I had better workouts in the gym, I did not get a dry mouth and I felt superb.

Eating salads and water along with the increase in training made me feel healthy and alive.

The best as I mentioned earlier, drinking water and fluids in between meals, ended my morning and afternoon cravings.

4

Chapter 3: The Role of Exercise

Nobody Said This Was Going to Be Easy

Embarking on a journey towards fitness is a commitment, and let's be honest – it's not a walk in the park. This chapter unravels the challenges and triumphs that come with integrating exercise into your lifestyle. From the essential role it plays in your transformation to the multitude of benefits it brings, this section is a testament to the resilience required to navigate the world of workouts.

The Benefits of Exercise

Exercise is more than just a means to burn calories it was for me, it was the key change that helped me to reshape my body without having to resort to cosmetic surgery or liposuction.

My exercise of choice was weightlifting. Weightlifting was something that I had done on and off over the years. In my younger days, I preferred martial arts as my choice of sport as opposed to weightlifting.

This was the fight of my life and I wanted to win this fight more than anything else in the world. I believe that if you are going to do something, you should do it properly. My aims were clear, lose the pot belly, make myself stronger, and say goodbye to my diagnosis.

Weight training gave me purpose and the motivation to keep going when I was feeling tired and sore. I picked myself up, dusted myself down, and through rain and shine, I went to the gym every day. I even on occasion, went to the gym in the mornings before work and in the evenings after my boys had gone to bed.

Weightlifting flicked a switch in me that had been dormant overtaken by life and children. Weight training unlocked my mental toughness, grit, and determination to succeed no matter what hurdles and challenges were thrown in front of me.

I reduced my waist size from 36 inches to 31 inches, my stomach is now flat and I can see my abdominal muscles when I look in the mirror. I was stronger, fitter, and leaner than I previously had been in my thirties. The reboot of myself had started.

I was sleeping like a baby and I had increased stamina. I thought I had peaked but I was wrong. For the first time in my existence, I was physically able to complete body-weight pull-ups in a neutral and wide grip.

Recording and Tracking Your Training

To track my progress in the gym, I purchased a smartwatch exercise tracker which came with an app. The app on my mobile telephone allowed me to record my workouts, my daily activity, and my sleeping patterns. In addition, I noted down every workout I completed including the weights I pushed and pulled and the repetitions in a notebook. The benefits I gained by tracking my training sessions allowed me to monitor my progress in real-time and gave me immediate gratification because I could see from my training results that I was training hard every session. I also had tangible evidence in my notebook that I was getting stronger and becoming fitter.

I soon had to invest in new clothing to wear at the gym because twelve weeks into my new regime, my old clothes did not fit me anymore. This was a blessing in disguise because I had to buy new training clothes, gym shoes, and accessories. My new gym clothing and accessories gave me even more motivation because after all, what is the point of buying new clothing, and accessories if you are not going to use them? The best example would be having all the tools and having no idea how to use them.

I remained motivated and resilient by doing things in the gymnasium properly such as warming up and warming down. Thankfully I did not pick up any injuries which allowed me to train every day. On occasion, I have to travel for my work. I always book a hotel that has a gym so that I can carry on working out even when I am away from home in another city.

The key to my weight training was focusing on different body parts on different days. For example, Monday was chest, Tuesday was arms and biceps, Wednesday was my back, Thursday was shoulders, and Friday was leg day. I found that by exercising the biggest muscles in my body, my legs, and training them hard, I obtained the most gains and got better results. I also incorporated full-body exercises on leg day so that I got the most gains by pushing my legs to their limits in the gym.

The consistency of working out every day got me into a rhythm. I went to bed early, I got up early and I rested when I needed to. My joints and bones felt great and still do. I felt re-born as if I had paused the sands of time.

I have carried on weight training because it not only gives me the most satisfaction, it also gives me the most bang for my buck in terms of results. Weight training is something I recommend to both men and women over the age of thirty. You are never too old and I think you would all enjoy it. I have embraced and accepted that weight training has helped me to unlock a healthier me.

5

Chapter 4: Fasting

So what is all of this Hullabaloo about Fasting and what is it?

Fasting can be defined in simple terms as a prolonged period of not eating food. For me personally fasting was and is the cornerstone of unlocking a healthier you. Let us look at prehistoric men and women, they did not have access to fast food, fizzy drinks, convenience, or grocery stores. They had to do things the hard way by hunting and catching their food. Only when they were successful during the hunt could they eat and feed each other provided that they were not eaten by bigger and better predators. Prehistoric men and women fasted for periods in between their hunts for food because they had no other choice.

For me, fasting is not only just as a means to reduce my body weight but fasting and weight training combined with a good diet including lots of salads and green vegetables reduced my blood sugars back to normal in seven months of dedicated training and fasting. Fasting for me personally has been superb, the benefits have been endless like a gift that keeps giving.

Fasting for me is the most powerful tool in my journey towards a healthier lifestyle and through fasting I unlocked the key to a healthier me. If it had not been for my diagnosis none of this would have happened. Every cloud has a silver lining.

The Different Types of Fasting

Fasting for me was never a and is not a one-size-fits-all approach. There are many different ways of fasting and many different terms used to describe fasting methods. My personal choice or rather the method of fasting that worked for me was one meal a day. I found that by not eating breakfast in the morning and not eating dinner in the evening worked. I relaxed the rules on weekends to accommodate family life and everything that comes with that. I discovered that it is possible to be lean and to be fit provided you were willing to commit.

The sweet spot for me was eating one meal a day which consisted of a large salad and green vegetables with nuts, eggs, and chicken at lunchtime.

I started by skipping breakfast, which was the easiest way to start my fasting journey. I was able to achieve this goal with ease. Skipping breakfast was not much of a big change in my lifestyle or eating habits because I often skipped breakfast in the mornings. The hardest part of my fasting journey was the initial sugar lust and cravings because I stopped eating sugary foods overnight.

To conquer the food cravings and sugar lust, I drank lots of water and black coffee in the mornings. In the afternoons after midday, I drank black decaffeinated coffee and water completely to counter the cravings. I missed eating sugary foods and drinking fizzy.

As I eased myself into fasting and fitness, I noticed the changes in my body after approximately four weeks. The quick turnaround from action to positive results blew my mind. By making subtle changes in my eating habits and could already see the light at the end of the tunnel. The visible changes spurred me on so much that I continue to this day with fasting and fitness. Fasting has been a master stroke for me and is something that I continue to do as I write this book.

At that moment I did not have to eat more than one meal a day provided I ate my loaded green vegetable salad at lunchtime, I was good to go for the rest of the day. My previous experience of attempting to lose weight was a strategy of eating small meals more often. Compared to fasting and fitness there was no contest. Eating one meal a day at lunchtime coupled with daily efforts in the gym boosted my energy, health, and turbocharged my results.

The Benefits of Fasting

I found that beyond weight loss, fasting unlocked a healthier me and provided me with a lean healthy body. My approach to fasting and fitness worked beyond my wildest expectations. Fasting for me is no longer a temporary fix, it is the solution.

Weekend Treats

While commitment is key, life is meant to be enjoyed. I employed a strategy of "Weekend Treats" and found that incorporating flexibility into my fasting routine contributed to a balanced and sustainable approach.

I fast from Monday to Friday and indulge in my favorite food and drinks at the weekend. When the weekend is over on a Monday morning it is back to business, back to Fasting and Fitness.

I enjoy and look forward to the weekend because I do not have to fast. The weekend is my prize for all of the hard work that I put in during the week. After all, all hard work and no play makes a boring man. I like to let my hair down and enjoy my weekends.

6

Conclusion

As I conclude my journey with you, my message to you all is that fasting and fitness worked for me. The results achieved were far better than I could ever have imagined and completely exceeded expectations.

I had won my battle thanks to my new routine of fasting and fitness. This was a war of mind over matter which I won because I was committed and went all in to achieve my goal of turning around my pre-diabetes diagnosis.

Life, with its demands and distractions, can make us forget how truly amazing we are. This book aims to serve as a reminder. You must never allow yourself to believe that you cannot do anything.

The only person who can stop you is you. We all have busy lives but you only get one life and you should live your best life possible.

Remember you can do anything with your life that you want to because you are a wonderful human being.

7

The final words

This book documents my own experience of being diagnosed as pre-diabetic in November through to being re-tested in the following June when my blood sugar was back to normal seven months later.

Disclaimer

I hope you the readers are inspired by what I did to overcome my health struggles.

Before attempting any new fasting and fitness regime, please speak to your doctor or physician so that they can carry out any relevant medical tests and examinations before you commence any new fasting and fitness regime.

I would recommend that you do not attempt any fitness and fasting regime until your doctor or physician has given you the green light to start.

www.ingramcontent.com/pod-product-compliance
Lightning Source LLC
Chambersburg PA
CBHW050759250726
48662CB00005B/2305